Debbie Martin

The Clever Guts Diet
Recipe Book

Contents

Chapter One - Breakfast Recipes

Chapter Two - Lunch Recipes

Chapter Three - Dinner Recipes

Chapter Four - Salad Recipes

Chapter Five - Soup Recipes

Chapter Six - Snack Recipes

Chapter Seven - Dessert Recipes

Introduction

Bacteria and other microbes (including fungi and viruses) are often thought of as sources of disease. However, while some undoubtedly are, the majority actually play an essential role in keeping us healthy.

Our bodies contains trillions of microbes (known collectively as known as the 'microbiome'), and most of them are found in the gut where they play a critical role in digestion, immune function and weight regulation.

Studies have demonstrated that these microbes reduce the incidence of a range of conditions. These include cancer, heart disease, liver disease, diabetes, asthma, depression, autism, irritable bowel syndrome, colic, Parkinson's disease and allergies of many types.

Unfortunately, most of us have a depleted microbiome because we are eating a poor diet that's high in sugar, refined carbohydrates, processed foods, artificial sweeteners and antibiotics.

This leads us to the purpose of this book. The recipes it offers are all formulated to not just prevent the depletion of good microbes but to actively foster their growth.

To this end, the recipes include a wide range of plant-based foods. This is critical because a healthy gut contains a diverse community of microbes, all of which thrive on different types of food. Furthermore, eating plant-based foods ensures an adequate intake of fibre, something most people eat much less of than they should.

Many of the recipes contain prebiotic foods that feed existing gut bacteria and encourage the growth of new ones.

The recipes also feature probiotic foods, such as live yoghurt, some cheeses and fermented foods. These actually contain live bacteria that are beneficial to the health of the gut.

A related issue that affects the majority of people in the western world is that of obesity - current figures suggest that two-thirds of us are overweight; many seriously so. Anyone who needs to lose weight will find that eating the gut-friendly recipes in this book will help them do so as surely as night follows day.

Breakfast Recipes

Shakshuka

Shakshuka is a Middle Eastern dish that can be eaten at breakfast, lunch or dinner. Packed with nutrients, I recommend it for breakfast as it will get your day off to the perfect start.

<u>**Serves 4**</u>

2 onions, sliced
225g spinach
2 red bell peppers, sliced
2 x 400g tins diced tomatoes
85g feta cheese
6 eggs
6 tbsp natural yoghurt
3 garlic cloves, finely chopped
2 tbsp olive oil
1 tsp chilli powder
1/2 tsp cumin seeds
1/2 tsp caraway seeds
1/4 tsp salt
Chopped parsley, for garnish

Heat the olive oil in a frying pan and cook the sliced onion and red pepper for 5 minutes. Then add the spinach and garlic and cook for 2 or 3 minutes more until the spinach has wilted. Add the cumin and caraway seeds, chilli powder and the diced tomatoes.

Without covering the pan, let the mixture simmer for

cont'd

10 minutes or so. Keep on eye on it as you don't want it to dry out - add some water if necessary.

When 10 minutes are up, make six wells in the sauce with a spoon. Then carefully break an egg into each well. Continue cooking until the whites of the eggs are just set.

Finished by crumbling the feta cheese and sprinkling it over the mixture.

Garnish with the chopped parsley and serve with yoghurt on the side.

Quesadilla

This breakfast quesadilla recipe is delicious. It's full of healthy fats that include almond butter and coconut oil. Another 'get-you-on-your-way' breakfast.

Serves 1

2 brown rice tortillas
1 peach, peeled and diced
25g almond butter
1/2 tbsp coconut oil
1/2 tbsp honey
Cinnamon to taste

Spread the almond butter on one tortilla and then put the diced peach on top. Drizzle the peach with the honey and then sprinkle with the cinnamon. Place the second tortilla on top.

In a frying pan over a medium heat, melt the coconut oil. Place the quesadilla in the pan and, flipping as necessary, cook it until both sides are golden brown and crispy.

Serve.

Bircher Muesli

Bircher muesli was first made over a century ago by the Swiss doctor Maximilian Bircher-Benner in his Zurich clinic. It is traditionally left overnight to soften the oats.

Serves 2

1 apple, coarsely grated
1 banana, sliced
100g full-fat yoghurt
50g porridge oats
25g sultanas
1 tsp mixed seeds
1 tsp mixed nuts, roughly chopped
1/2 tsp ground cinnamon

Put the grated apple in a bowl and add the oats, seeds, half the nuts and the cinnamon. Toss together well.

Stir in the yoghurt and 100ml of cold water, cover and chill for several hours or overnight.

Spoon the muesli into two bowls and top with the sliced banana, sultanas and remaining nuts.

Scrambled Egg With Asparagus

The key to making scrambled eggs is whisking the eggs thoroughly before cooking them. This adds air, which makes them lighter and fluffier.

Serves 2

4 eggs
100g asparagus spears
1 mushroom
1 tomato
2 slices of ham
50ml milk
2 tsp butter
Small handful of chopped tarragon or chervil
Slices of ciabatta, warmed

Steam the asparagus spears for 4-5 mins until tender.

Place the eggs and milk in a bowl and whisk to a smooth consistency. Chop the tomato, mushroom and ham as finely as you can and stir them into the egg mixture.

Melt the butter in a frying pan and then add the egg mixture. With the pan on a medium heat, slowly cook it, stirring continuously.

When the scrambled egg is firm, pile it on to the asparagus and hot, buttered slices of ciabatta. Top with a few shavings of parmesan if desired and serve.

Salmon Kedgeree

This version of the breakfast classic is made with fresh salmon instead of smoked haddock, which is high in salt; and cauliflower instead of rice, which is high in carbohydrates.

<u>Serves 2</u>

1/2 cauliflower, grated
2 eggs
1 onion, finely chopped
150g salmon
150ml milk
2 tsp olive oil
1 tbsp yoghurt
1 lemon, juice of
2 tbsp cumin, finely chopped

Hard boil the eggs for 15 minutes, shell and cut them into quarters. Put the grated cauliflower into a pan together with the milk and simmer for 5 minutes. Drain and put to one side.

Heat the olive oil in a frying pan and fry the onion for 5 minutes. Add the salmon and cook for another 5 minutes. Then add the lemon juice, yoghurt and cumin and mix thoroughly.

Finally, combine the cauliflower with the salmon/ vegetable mixture and top with the quartered eggs.

Mushroom Quiche

The secret of this quiche is that it doesn't contain any pastry, i.e. carbohydrates.

Serves 4

300g mushrooms, chopped
150g cooked ham or bacon, diced
4 eggs
1 onion, finely chopped
200g cream cheese
100g cheddar cheese, grated
50g butter
2 tbsp breadcrumbs
2 tbsp parmesan cheese, grated
1/2 tsp black pepper, ground
Dash of tabasco sauce

In a pan, cook the mushrooms and onion in the butter until just tender - about 5 minutes. Then stir in the breadcrumbs, parmesan cheese and pepper.

Butter the bottom and sides of a pie dish. Press the mushroom mixture into the dish. Sprinkle the grated cheddar on top of it.

In a blender, beat the cream cheese, eggs and Tabasco sauce together until well mixed. Stir in the diced ham. Then pour the mixture over the mushrooms and cheese in the baking dish. Bake for 30 minutes.

Baked Eggs With Spinach

A hearty one-pot meal with a delicious combination of flavours. For a meatier dish, add chunks of cooked chicken, ham or bacon when you add the eggs.

<u>Serves 4</u>

200g new potatoes, thickly sliced
1 onion, finely chopped
1/2 bell pepper, de-seeded and chopped
1 x 200g tin cannellini beans
4 eggs
2 tomatoes, chopped
50g spinach
150ml passata
1 tbsp Worcestershire sauce
1 garlic clove, chopped
Handful of oregano

Boil the potatoes in a pan until they are tender and then drain them. Next, fry the onion, garlic and pepper in a frying pan for 5 minutes.

Add them all to a large pan together with the beans, tomatoes, passata and Worcestershire sauce. Season and simmer for 10-12 minutes.

Stir in the spinach. Then make four wells in the mixture and crack an egg into each one. Cover and cook for 5 minutes. Finally, garnish with the oregano.

Creamy Yoghurt Porridge

This delicious oaty breakfast is low in fat and calories but high in gut-friendly fibre. It is also a balanced source of protein, fats, carbohydrates, vitamins and minerals from the probiotic yoghurt.

Serves 2

150g pot Greek yoghurt
300ml milk
50g porridge oats
2 tbsp raisins

Pour the milk into a small pan and stir in the porridge oats.

Cook over a low heat until the oats are bubbling and have thickened. Add more milk or oats as necessary to achieve the desired thickness.

Stir in the yoghurt and then top with the raisins.

Serve.

French Omelette

Chock-full of healthy ingredients, this omelette will get your day off to a great start.

<u>Serves 1</u>

1 mushroom, finely diced
1 tomato, chopped
1 onion
1 clove garlic, minced
2 eggs
25g mozzarella cheese
1 tsp basil
1 tbsp olive oil

Put the eggs and the basil in a bowl and whisk to a frothy consistency. Put to one side.

Then put the mushrooms, onion and garlic in a frying pan and fry them in the olive oil until cooked.

Add the egg and basil mixture to the frying pan over a medium heat and cook the omelette until it has set.

Sprinkle the mozzarella cheese over it, add the chopped tomato and serve.

Cinnamon Granola Bars

These granola bars are great for lunch boxes, breakfast on the run or just with a cup of coffee.

Makes 10

200g porridge oats
100g mixed berries
100g butter
50g sunflower seeds
50g sesame seeds
50g walnuts, chopped
1 tsp honey
1 tsp cinnamon

Preheat the oven to 160°C, gas mark 3.

Butter and line the base of a medium size baking tin.

Mix the oats, seeds and walnuts in a roasting tin and then put them in the oven for 5-10 minutes to toast.

Next, melt the butter and honey in a pan. Add the oat mix, cinnamon and mixed berries, then mix until it is all well coated with the butter and honey.

Tip into the baking tin, compact the mixture lightly and then bake it for 30 minutes.

Allow to cool in the tin before cutting into ten bars.

Applesauce Pancakes

These delicious grain-free applesauce pancakes are not only a high-protein breakfast option but are also gluten-free.

<u>Makes 5</u>

2 eggs
55g almond flour
5 tbsp unsweetened applesauce
1/2 tsp baking powder
1/4 tsp vanilla extract
1/2 tbsp maple syrup
1 tbsp olive oil

First, whisk the two eggs in a small bowl. Then add the applesauce, maple syrup and vanilla extract.

Next, add the almond flour and baking powder, and mix thoroughly to make a batter

Heat the olive oil in a frying pan. Then spoon in about 3 tablespoons of the batter. Let it cook until firm enough to flip - about 3-4 minutes.

Cook the second side for around 2-3 minutes. Repeat until all the batter has been used.

Egg & Leek Bake

This hearty country dish from the Provence region of France is an easy mix of seasonal vegetables, garlic and olive oil.

<u>Serves 2</u>

3 eggs
1 leek, thinly sliced
100g mushrooms, sliced
2 tbsp yoghurt
Pinch of black pepper
1 tsp olive oil

Preheat the oven to 170°C, gas mark 4.

Put the olive oil in a frying pan and add the sliced leek and mushrooms. Stirring regularly, cook for 5 minutes.

Then mix in the yoghurt and black pepper. When done, place the mixture in an oven-proof dish and bake for 15 minutes.

Remove from the oven and serve.

Almond Granola

This homemade granola is a healthier version of the shop-bought varieties, which are almost always much higher in sugar.

<u>**Serves 2**</u>

250g oats
100g apricots, chopped
1 egg
40g almonds, flaked
50g raisins
2 tsp of honey
1 tsp olive oil

Preheat the oven to 150°C, gas mark 2.

Put the oats and almonds in a bowl and mix well.

In a separate bowl, beat the egg together with the honey until a frothy consistency has been achieved. Then add the oats and almonds and combine thoroughly.

Grease a baking sheet with the olive oil. Spread the mixture onto the baking sheet, place it in the oven and bake for about 15 minutes. Finally, add the raisins and apricots and bake for 10 more minutes.

Remove from the oven and serve.

Apple & Cinnamon Bowl

Packed with nutritional goodness, this is a light, energizing and satisfying breakfast that will power you through the morning.

<u>Serves 2</u>

3 apples, peeled and cored
4 medjool dates, pitted
2 tbsp chia seeds
1/2 tsp ground cinnamon
1/2 tsp nutmeg

Topping:
1 tbsp walnuts
1 tbsp raisins
1 tbsp dried cranberries

Chop the apples into large pieces and then add them to a food processor along with the dates, cinnamon and nutmeg. Blitz the ingredients until thoroughly combined.

Put the mixture into two bowls and top with the walnuts, raisins and dried cranberries.

Serve.

Lunch Recipes

Chicken & Banana Sambal

This spicy Asian-inspired dish is flavoured with coriander, cumin, turmeric, almonds and cardamom. Serve with a cooling chopped salad.

Serves 6

500g chicken breast, cut into chunks
2 onions, chopped
500ml chicken stock
1 chilli pepper, finely chopped
4 garlic cloves
2.5cm root ginger, chopped
1 tsp ground coriander
1 tsp ground cumin
1/2 tsp ground turmeric
2 tbsp ground almond
2 tbsp tomato purée
Small handful coriander, chopped

For the sambal and rice:
1 small onion, finely chopped
1/4 cucumber, diced
1 banana, diced
1/2 lime, zest and juice of
250g pack ready-cooked brown basmati rice

Put the onions in a food processor with the garlic and ginger. Blitz until it is as smooth as possible then pour in half the chicken stock and blitz again.

cont'd

Heat a large non-stick pan, sprinkle in the spices and toast for 1 minute. Pour in the onion mixture, the remaining stock and all but half a teaspoon of the chopped chilli. Add the almonds and tomato purée, and stir well.

Simmer for 35 minutes until completely soft, stirring occasionally and adding a little water if necessary.

Add the chicken and half the coriander. Heat very gently for 10 minutes to cook the chicken through.

Mix all the sambal ingredients with the remaining coriander and chilli, and heat the rice following the instructions on the pack.

Serve the chicken and sambal with the brown rice.

Pancetta Greens

This is a great way to get your greens! You can use different greens than those specified below depending on what's in season.

Serves 2

1 x 400g tin cannellini beans, drained
2 slices pancetta or bacon, chopped
1 onion, chopped
1 tbsp olive oil
Bunch of kale, chopped
Bunch of beet greens, chopped
3 cloves garlic, crushed
Salt and pepper

In a frying pan, heat the olive oil over a medium heat. Add the pancetta and cook until done. Remove from the pan and put to one side.

Now cook the onion in the same oil (add more if there's not enough left from the pancetta). Then add the crushed garlic cloves and cook one minute more. Stir in the chopped kale and beet greens, and season with salt and pepper to taste.

Cook until the greens begin to wilt. Then stir in the pancetta and cannellini beans and cook for 5 more minutes to allow the flavours to combine.

Then serve.

Quinoa Pilaf

This creamy pilaf combines fluffy, nutty-flavoured quinoa with cheese to give a most unusual flavour and texture.

<u>Serves 1</u>

4 tbsp quinoa
3 tbsp olive oil
2 tbsp sunflower seeds
2 cloves garlic, minced
50g spinach leaves
2 tsp lemon juice
25g cheddar, grated

Bring a pot of lightly salted water to the boil. Add the quinoa and cook until it is soft. Drain and set aside.

Heat the olive oil in a frying pan, stir in the sunflower seeds and cook for about 2 minutes until lightly toasted. Stir in the garlic and cook for 2 more minutes.

Next in is the cooled quinoa and spinach leaves - stir until the quinoa is hot and the spinach has wilted.

Finally, add the lemon juice and all but a pinch of the cheese. Stir until the cheese has melted. Serve the pilaf with the remaining cheese sprinkled on top.

Grilled Avocado Salmon

This dish provides a practical and delicious option for barbecues and lunches.

Serves 4

1kg salmon steak
2 avocados, pitted and diced
3 tbsp yoghurt
2 cloves garlic, crushed
1 tbsp lemon juice
2 tsp dried dill
Salt and pepper to taste

In a medium sized bowl, mash together the avocados, garlic, yoghurt and lemon juice. Season the mixture with salt and pepper.

Rub the salmon with the dill, lemon juice, pepper and salt. Place it under a preheated grill (an outdoor grill is highly recommended if available), and cook for 15 minutes, turning as necessary until cooked right through.

Serve with the avocado mixture.

Ginger & Vegetable Stir Fry

An extremely healthy dish with a mild ginger flavour that is filling yet light on the tummy.

1 onion, chopped
1 head broccoli, cut into florets
75g green peas
1 carrot, chopped
5cm root ginger, chopped
1 tbsp cornstarch
1 clove garlic, crushed
4 tbsp olive oil
2 tbsp soy sauce
2 tbsp water

In a bowl, mix the cornstarch with the garlic, half the ginger and 2 tbsp of olive oil until it has dissolved. Then mix in the broccoli, peas and carrots, tossing so they are lightly coated with the mixture.

Heat the remaining 2 tbsp of olive oil in a frying pan over a medium heat. Cook the vegetables in the oil for 2 minutes, stirring continuously.

Stir in the soy sauce and water. Finally, add the onion, salt and the rest of the ginger. Cook until the vegetables are tender.

Black Bean Burgers

Very easy and quick to make, these vegetarian burgers are not only delicious, they're also extremely good for you.

<u>Makes 4</u>

1 x 400g tin black beans, drained and rinsed
1/2 bell pepper, chopped
1 small onion, chopped
1 egg
100g bread crumbs
3 cloves garlic
1 tsp chilli powder
1 tsp hot sauce

Put the beans in a bowl and mash them with a fork until thick and pasty.

Using a food processor, finely chop the bell pepper, onion and garlic. Then stir into the mashed beans.

In a bowl, mix the egg, chilli powder and chilli sauce. Add the mixture to the beans and stir until it is well combined. Now add the bread crumbs and stir until the mixture is sticky enough to hold together.

Divide it into four patties. Place the patties on a preheated grill and grill each side for about 8 minutes.

Chicken Piccata

Chicken Piccata is a classic and comforting Italian dish made with, amongst other things, lemon, butter and white wine.

<u>Serves 4</u>

4 chicken breasts
1 x 200g tin artichoke hearts, drained and chopped
1 onion, diced
150g white flour
1 clove garlic, diced
2 tbsp olive oil
150ml white wine
1/4 tsp garlic powder
1/2 tsp Italian seasoning
2 tbsp lemon juice
2 tbsp butter

In a bowl, mix together the flour, garlic powder and Italian seasoning. Then coat the chicken pieces lightly in the mixture.

Heat the olive oil in a pan over a medium to high heat and cook the chicken halves for 2 minutes per side, or until nicely browned. Remove from the pan and set aside.

Using the same pan, now cook the garlic and onion for 5 minutes or so. Add the lemon juice, white wine,

cont'd

artichoke hearts and coated chicken to the pan.

Reduce the heat to low and cook for about 20 minutes until a thick sauce has been created. Stir in the butter and serve.

Chickpeas & Chilli

Tender cooked chickpeas are simmered lightly with tomatoes, lemon juice and onions in a spicy blend of toasted cumin seeds and chilli powder.

<u>Serves 2</u>

1 onion, chopped
1 tomato, chopped
200g chickpeas
1 tbsp olive oil
1 tsp cumin seeds
1/2 tsp salt
1/2 tsp chilli powder
1 tbsp lemon juice

Heat the cumin seeds in the olive oil until they turn a dark shade of brown.

Add the salt and chilli powder, and mix well. Stir in the chopped tomato and, when the juice begins to thicken, add the chickpeas and mix thoroughly.

Finally, add the onion and lemon juice. Cook until the onion is soft. Remove from the heat and serve immediately.

Red Lentil & Bean Curry

A very tasty vegetarian curry that you will just love. Serve with rice or on naan bread.

Serves 4

225g red lentils
225g plain yoghurt
2 tomatoes, chopped
1 x 400g tin mixed beans, rinsed and drained
1 onion, chopped
50g tomato puree
2 cloves garlic, chopped
2.5cm root ginger, grated
1 tsp garam masala
1/2 tsp of turmeric
1/2 tsp cumin
2 tbsp olive oil
4 sprigs fresh coriander, chopped

Rinse the lentils and place them in a saucepan with enough water to cover. Bring to the boil and then reduce the heat to low. Cover the saucepan and let the lentils cook over a low heat for 20 minutes. Remove them from the pan and drain.

In a bowl, mix the tomato puree and yoghurt. Season with garam masala, turmeric and cumin. Stir until a creamy consistency has been achieved.

cont'd

Heat the olive oil in a pan over a medium heat. Stir in the onion, garlic and ginger, and cook until the onion begins to brown.

Now gradually stir in the yoghurt and tomato puree mixture. Then add the tomatoes and coriander.

Finally, add the cooked lentils and mixed beans to the mixture and stir until well combined.

Heat to the desired temperature and then serve.

Kimchi Pancakes

These spicy Korean-style pancakes make a quick and nutrient-rich lunch that is also extremely appetising.

Makes 2

225g kimchi
225g flour
2 eggs
1 onion, finely chopped
1 tbsp olive oil
1 tbsp rice vinegar
1 tbsp soy sauce
1/2 tbsp sesame oil
1 tsp sesame seeds

Make the batter by blitzing the kimchi (including the juice), flour, eggs and onion in a food processor.

Heat the olive oil over a medium heat in a frying pan. Then pour half of the batter into the pan, spreading as thinly as possible. Cook the pancake on each side until it has set and is lightly browned. Repeat with the remainder of the batter to make the second pancake.

Whisk together the rice vinegar, soy sauce, sesame oil and sesame seeds. Serve with the pancakes.

Cauliflower Rice

This low calorie meal is perfect for a quick lunch. Rather than use carbohydrate-high rice though, the recipe uses grated cauliflower as a healthier substitute.

<u>Serves 2</u>

1 x 225g tin bamboo shoots, drained
1/2 cauliflower, grated
70g peas
1 onion, finely chopped
1/2 bell pepper, chopped
70g pineapple, cut into small chunks
100g prawns
2 tsp olive oil
2 tbsp Thai green curry paste
150ml milk

Heat the olive oil in a frying pan and fry the onion for 5 minutes. Stir in the pepper, pineapple and the green curry paste and cook for 3 more minutes.

Put the cauliflower in a pan with the milk and simmer it for 5 minutes. Then drain the milk and return the cauliflower to the pan.

Stir the peas, bamboo shoots and prawns into the 'cauliflower rice', then cook for 2 or 3 minutes until the prawns are hot and the peas tender. Then add the onion and pepper mixture, stir well and serve.

Collard Greens & Cannellini Beans

This is a simple recipe for collard greens that is easy and fast.

1 x 400g tin cannellini beans, rinsed and drained
225g collard greens, chopped
2 tomatoes, chopped
2 onions, chopped
2 cloves garlic, minced
1 cube beef-flavoured bouillon
2 tbsp water, or more as needed
Salt and pepper

Heat the 2 tablespoons of water in a large pan over a medium heat. Cook the onion and garlic in the water for about 5 minutes, adding more water as needed to prevent scorching. Stir the bouillon cube into the onion and garlic mixture.

Stir the collard greens and tomatoes (and more water if necessary) into the mixture. Cover and let it simmer for about 20 minutes until the vegetables are nice and tender.

Now add the cannellini beans and continue simmering until all the liquid has evaporated.

Season to taste and serve.

Chicken with Black Beans

Seared strips of chicken with crunchy bamboo shoots and water chestnuts in a savoury black bean sauce. A very popular dish in China and Malaysia.

Serves 4

1 x 400g tin black beans, drained
1 onion, finely chopped
800g of chicken breasts, cut into strips
1 large carrot, chopped into strips
1 bell pepper, chopped
5 spring onions, cut into strips
1 x 225g tin bamboo shoots, drained
1 x 225g tin sliced water chestnuts, drained
400ml chicken stock
2.5cm root ginger, finely chopped
3 garlic cloves, finely chopped
2 tsp Marmite
3 tbsp olive oil
3 tbsp light soy sauce

Put the ginger, garlic, Marmite and half the black beans into a food processor and blend to a smooth paste, adding a little water if necessary.

Heat 1 tbsp of olive oil in a frying pan over a medium heat. Add the onion and fry it for 5 minutes. Stir in the black bean paste, soy sauce, 300ml of the stock and the remaining black beans and simmer until

cont'd

thickened. Remove from the pan and set aside.

Next, place another frying pan (or wok) over a medium heat. Add another 1 tbsp of olive oil and cook the chicken for 6-7 minutes. When done, transfer the chicken to a plate.

With the final 1 tbsp of olive oil, stir-fry the carrot and red pepper for 3 minutes. Add the spring onions, bamboo shoots and water chestnuts and cook for another 2 minutes.

Finally, add the chicken and the black bean sauce to the wok along with the remaining stock, season with pepper and bring to a simmer.

After 5 minutes of simmering, the dish will be ready to serve.

Bacon Quiche

Quick to make and nutrient-rich, this crustless quiche is ideal for lunch or a picnic when you're out and about.

Serves 4

220g lean bacon, cut into fine pieces
150g mushrooms, sliced
3 eggs
200g cottage cheese
4 cherry tomatoes, halved
2 garlic cloves, diced
2 tbsp chopped fresh parsley
Salt and pepper

Preheat the oven to 190°C, gas mark 5.

Fry the bacon for a couple of minutes before adding the mushrooms and garlic. Add seasoning as desired and continue to cook for about 5 minutes. Then put the mixture into a flan dish.

Mix the eggs, cottage cheese and parsley in a bowl and then ladle it over the bacon mixture.

Top with the tomato halves and bake in the oven for 15-20 minutes until set.

Thai Chilli Satay

This recipe uses Shirataki noodles, which are also known as 'miracle noodles', due to their very low carbohydrate content.

Serves 4

300g pack mixed stir-fry vegetables
300g Shirataki noodles
3 tbsp crunchy peanut butter
2.5cm root ginger, grated
3 tbsp sweet chilli sauce
2 tbsp soy sauce
1 tbsp olive oil
Handful of basil leaves

Mix the peanut butter, chilli sauce, 100ml of water and the soy sauce to make a smooth satay sauce. Put the noodles in a bowl and pour boiling water over them. Stir gently to separate, then drain thoroughly.

Heat the oil in a frying pan or wok, then stir-fry the ginger and harder pieces of veg from the stir-fry mix, such as peppers, for 2 minutes. Add the noodles and the rest of the vegetables, then stir-fry over a high heat for 1-2 minutes until the vegetables are cooked.

Add the satay sauce to the pan and mix with the vegetables and noodles. Cook until hot then place on serving plates. Garnish with the basil leaves to finish.

Courgette Quiche

This versatile vegetable quiche is not only healthy, it is ideal for lunch, dinner or informal entertaining.

<u>Serves 4</u>

1 onion, sliced
1 courgette, sliced
1 bell pepper, finely chopped
6 eggs
100g cheddar cheese, grated
2 tbsp tomato purée
2 tbsp olive oil
1 garlic clove, crushed
1 tbsp mixed herbs
Salt and pepper

Preheat the oven to 180°C, gas mark 4.

Put 1 tbsp of olive oil in a frying pan and cook the onions until they are lightly browned. Then transfer them to a wide bowl and put to one side.

Wipe the frying pan with kitchen paper to clean it and then add the remaining olive oil. Place over a medium heat, add the courgette and pepper and stir-fry for about 10 minutes until cooked. Remove from the pan and add to the bowl containing the onions.

Beat the eggs with the garlic, tomato purée, mixed

cont'd

herbs and three quarters of the cheese. Season well.

Put the onions, courgettes and red peppers in an oven-proof dish and pour the egg mixture on top. Bake in the oven for 40-45 minutes until almost set.

Remove the dish from the oven, sprinkle the remaining cheese on top and then return it to the oven. Bake until the quiche is lightly browned on top and just set.

Dinner Recipes

Curried Chicken Drumsticks

A quick, simple chicken curry that takes no time at all to prepare but tastes great.

<u>Serves 4</u>

8 chicken drumsticks
150g yoghurt
1 tbsp curry powder
5 tbsp coriander, chopped
5 tbsp mint, chopped
1 tsp turmeric
1 lime, zest and juice of
Salt and pepper

Place all the ingredients, apart from the chicken, in a food processor and blend until smooth. Transfer the marinade mixture to a large bowl.

Using a fork, pierce each drumstick all over in preparation for marinading. Place the drumsticks in the marinade and rub the marinade well into the chicken.

Remove the drumsticks from the marinade and grill them for about 20 minutes, turning occasionally, until cooked through. Serve warm or cold.

Venison Stir-Fry

Venison is a lovely, tasty meat. It also has half the calories and just one sixth of the amount of saturated fat found in beef. Try it with this delicious stir-fry.

<u>Serves 2</u>

300g venison, cut into thin strips
8 cherry tomatoes
1 leek, cut into strips
1/2 bell pepper, sliced
3 tbsp olive oil
3 tbsp sweet chilli sauce
2 tbsp sesame oil
1 tbsp soy sauce
Salt and pepper

Heat 1 tbsp of sesame oil in a frying pan and stir-fry the tomatoes for two minutes. Then add the venison, leek and pepper, and stir-fry for a further 5 minutes.

Next, pour the soy sauce into the pan, mix well and cook for another 3 minutes. Season with salt and pepper to taste.

Mix the sweet chilli sauce, olive oil and 1 tbsp of sesame oil in a small bowl to make a dressing.

Drizzle the venison stir-fry with the dressing and serve.

Jollof Chicken Rice

A popular West African dish that's cooked in one pan and is ideal for a simple, quick and tasty dinner.

Serves 4

350g chicken breast, cut into chunks
1 red bell pepper, chopped
1 yellow bell pepper, chopped
400g dry Shirataki rice
1 large onion, chopped
1 x 400g tin chopped tomatoes
100g okra, cut into 2cm pieces
2 garlic cloves, crushed
2.5cm root ginger, finely chopped
1 Scotch Bonnet chilli pepper, chopped
2 tbsp tomato purée
1 chicken stock cube dissolved in 450ml water
1 tbsp olive oil
2 tbsp chopped coriander

Heat the olive oil in a frying pan then add the onion and cook for 3-4 minutes until it's starting to brown.

Add the chicken chunks and cook for a further 3-4 minutes, stirring regularly to make sure the chicken is cooked evenly on all sides.

Next into the frying pan are the peppers. Carry on cooking for another 2 minutes or so before adding the

cont'd

garlic, ginger, chilli and tomato puree. Mix thoroughly and then add the rice, chicken stock and tomatoes. Bring to the boil, reduce the heat, cover and simmer for about 10 minutes.

Scatter the okra on top of the rice, replace the lid and simmer for a further 5 minutes.

Now turn off the heat but don't remove the lid. Leave to stand for 5 minutes. Add the coriander, give it one last stir and serve.

Note: Shirataki rice and noodles are both made from the root of a plant called Konnyaku. As they are made from the soluble fibre of the plant, they are extremely low in calories.

Butternut Squash Casserole

A warming seasonal dish with a fusion of flavours that is ideal for winter evenings.

Serves 6

225g sweet potato, cut into chunks
1 bell pepper, chopped
1 butternut squash, chopped
1 x 400g tin chopped tomatoes
1 onion, sliced
200ml red wine
300ml vegetable stock
75g bulgur wheat
4 tbsp Greek yoghurt
2 tbsp olive oil
2 garlic cloves, crushed
1 tsp cumin seeds

Heat the olive oil in a pan and cook the onion and garlic for 5 minutes. Add the cumin seeds, the sweet potato, red pepper and butternut squash, and cook for 2 minutes more.

Pour in the tomatoes, red wine and vegetable stock and simmer for 15 minutes. Stir in the bulgur wheat, cover with a lid, then simmer for another 15 minutes until the liquid has been absorbed.

Serve in bowls topped with the yoghurt.

Prawn Biryani

A fragrantly spiced pilaf-style dish that is extremely healthy. The recipe uses grated cauliflower instead of rice.

<u>Serves 4</u>

1/2 cauliflower, grated
300g baby leaf spinach, chopped
1 x 400g tin chopped tomatoes
1 onion, diced
1 red chilli pepper, finely chopped
225g peeled tiger prawns
1cm root ginger, grated
2 tbsp olive oil
1 tbsp ground cumin
1 tbsp ground coriander
1 tsp ground turmeric
1/2 tsp ground nutmeg
Pinch of sugar

Sieve the tomatoes, place them in a bowl and put to one side. Keep the sieved tomato juice as well.

Put a kettle of water on to boil.

Heat the olive oil in a large casserole dish over a medium heat. Add the onion, chilli and ginger, and stir for 3 minutes.

Stir in the cumin, coriander, turmeric and nutmeg,

cont'd

and continue stirring until the onion is cooked.

Add the grated cauliflower and drained tomatoes to the casserole and stir to mix with the spices. Add enough boiling water to the reserved tomato juice to make up to 450ml. Stir this liquid and the sugar into the casserole, add a pinch of salt, then bring to the boil.

Reduce the heat to low, cover tightly and leave the 'cauliflower rice' to cook without lifting the lid for 10–12 minutes.

Then stir in the spinach in small batches, adding more as each addition wilts. When all the spinach has been added, lay the prawns on top, re-cover the casserole and turn the heat down to very low.

Cook for 2 minutes, then turn off the heat and leave the casserole to stand for 1 minute, without lifting the lid. By this time the spinach will have wilted further and the prawns will have cooked through. Gently fork together to combine the cauliflower rice, spinach and prawns and then serve.

Beef & Red Wine Casserole

Tender beef and tasty vegetables cooked in a delicious red wine sauce make a dinner to remember.

<u>Serves 4</u>

800g lean stewing beef cut into chunks
2 carrots, chopped
2 leeks, sliced
4 celery sticks, cut into large pieces
1 x 400g tin chopped tomatoes with herbs
800ml beef stock
100ml red wine
3 garlic cloves, chopped
2 tsp dried mixed herbs
Salt and pepper

Preheat the oven to 180°C, gas mark 4.

Put the beef in a casserole dish together with the garlic, carrots, leeks and celery.

Stir in the beef stock, wine, tomatoes and the mixed herbs. Then bring the mixture to the boil over a high heat.

Cover the casserole dish, place it in the oven and cook for 2½ hours.

Then serve.

Caribbean Pepperpot Stew

Originating in Jamaica, this classic stew is hot, spicy and absolutely delicious.

Serves 4

800g lean stewing beef, cut into chunks
2 bell peppers, chopped
1 sweet potato, chopped
250g green beans, trimmed and halved
400g passata with onions and garlic
400ml beef stock
2 garlic cloves, finely chopped
2 tbsp jerk seasoning
1 tbsp red wine vinegar
2 tbsp Worcestershire sauce

Fry the beef in a pan for 5 minutes or so until cooked through. Then transfer it to a casserole dish and add the peppers, sweet potato, beans, garlic, jerk seasoning, wine vinegar, passata, beef stock and Worcestershire sauce. Mix thoroughly.

Put the dish in the oven at 180°C, gas mark 4, and cook for 2 hours.

The stew can be eaten on its own or with rice.

Tandoori Chicken

A favourite not just in India, but now in the UK as well. Spicy, easy to cook and very good for you.

Serves 4

8 chicken thighs
1 onion, finely chopped
1 lemon, juice of
2 tsp paprika
1 tsp olive oil

For the marinade:
300ml Greek yoghurt
2.5cm root ginger, grated
2 garlic cloves, crushed
1/2 tsp garam masala
1/2 tsp ground cumin
1/2 tsp turmeric

Mix the lemon juice with the paprika and onion in a large shallow dish. Slash the chicken thighs then turn them in the juice and put to one side.

Mix the marinade ingredients in a bowl and pour it over the chicken. Cover and chill for at least one hour.

Place the chicken pieces onto a hot grill. Brush with a little olive oil and grill until lightly charred and completely cooked through. Serve.

Vegetable Hotpot

A hearty one-pot dish of tender root vegetables cooked in a tomato-based stock.

Serves 4

2 x 400g tins chopped tomatoes
300g button mushrooms
1 onion, chopped
4 celery sticks, sliced
3 turnips, chopped
2 carrots, chopped
2 parsnips, chopped
3 potatoes, cut into chunks
60g yellow split peas
500ml vegetable stock
2 garlic cloves, diced
2 sprigs of rosemary

Place the onion, celery and half of the stock in a large saucepan. Bring to the boil, reduce the heat and simmer for 10 minutes.

Add the remaining stock with the garlic, turnips, carrots, parsnips and potatoes. Bring back to the boil and add the split peas, tomatoes and mushrooms.

Bring the mixture back to the boil once again, reduce the heat, season well and simmer gently for about 20 minutes until the vegetables are tender. Serve.

Cheese & Onion Pie

Mashed potato mixed with finely diced vegetables, topped with grated cheddar cheese, then baked in the oven - a simple yet satisfying dish.

<u>Serves 4</u>

3 medium potatoes, chopped
3 onions, chopped
1 carrot, chopped
100g green beans, trimmed and diced
3 eggs
4 tsp dried parsley
200g cottage cheese
120g cheddar cheese, grated
2 tbsp olive oil

Preheat the oven to 180°C, gas mark 5.

Cook the potatoes by bringing them to the boil in a in a saucepan, then reducing the heat and simmering for 20-25 minutes.

While the potatoes are cooking, boil the carrot and green beans in a saucepan of lightly salted boiling water for 3-4 minutes. Drain and put to one side.

Put 1 tbsp of olive oil in a pan and place over a medium-high heat. Add the onions and stir-fry until nicely browned.

cont'd

When the potatoes are ready, drain them and then mash until smooth. Put to one side.

Now, in a small bowl, whisk together the eggs, dried parsley and cottage cheese. Add to the potatoes, stir to mix well and season to taste. Add the vegetables and onion to the potatoes and stir well again.

Brush the inside of a medium-sized pie dish with the rest of the olive oil.

Transfer the mixture to the pie dish and spread it out evenly. Sprinkle the cheese on top and bake for about 40 minutes.

Sprinkle with the chopped parsley and serve.

Pepper Ciambotta

Ciambotta is a vegetable stew, the ingredients of which can vary according to what's on hand. It makes a delicious accompaniment to roasted chicken, fish or meat.

<u>Serves 4</u>

1 bell pepper, chopped
1 x 400g tin tomatoes
2 medium courgettes, chopped
200g green beans, chopped
1 onion, chopped
2 bulbs of fennel
2 cloves of garlic, diced
2 tbsp olive oil
Handful of basil leaves

Heat the olive oil over a medium heat and then add the onion and fennel. Cook for 5 minutes until they are lightly browned and tender. Add the pepper and garlic, and cook for another 5 minutes or so.

Add the tomatoes (with the juice), the courgettes and green beans. Raise the heat to medium-high, stirring and breaking up the tomatoes. Then reduce the heat to medium-low, cover, and simmer for 25-30 minutes until all the vegetables are tender.

Top with the basil and serve.

Onion Frittata

A traditional and popular dish in Italy, this delicious frittata is a quick and tasty dinner.

<u>Serves 4</u>

3 onions, chopped
100g cherry tomatoes, halved
4 spring onions, finely diced
120g parmesan cheese, grated
4 eggs
250g quark
2 tbsp balsamic vinegar
Small handful of thyme leaves, chopped

Preheat the oven to 160°C, gas mark 3.

Lightly grease the inside of an over-proof dish and then add the onions, cherry tomatoes and balsamic vinegar. Mix the ingredients before placing the dish in the oven for 10 minutes or so. Then remove it from the oven and put it to one side.

In a bowl, whisk the quark and eggs. Add the thyme, season to taste, and stir in the diced spring onions. Pour this mixture into the dish and mix well. Sprinkle the grated parmesan cheese on top.

Return the dish to the oven and bake for 35-40 minutes. Remove and serve.

Prawn Dhansak

Filling lentils are at the heart of this colourful curry flavoured with mild spices, garlic and ginger.

Serves 2

2 shallots, thinly sliced
2 bell peppers, roughly chopped
1 x 400g tin lentils, drained and rinsed
4 cherry tomatoes, halved
100g peeled prawns
50g baby spinach leaves
2 garlic cloves, crushed
1cm piece root ginger, grated
1 tsp tandoori curry powder
100ml vegetable stock
1 tbsp olive oil
1 lemon, cut into wedges

Heat the olive oil in a saucepan and then cook the shallots and peppers for 3-4 minutes. Add the garlic, ginger and tandoori curry powder and cook for a further 1-2 minutes.

Next, add the lentils, tomatoes and vegetable stock, bring to the boil then reduce the heat to low and let it simmer for 4-5 minutes. Add the prawns and spinach, then cover and cook for 5 minutes.

Serve with the lemon wedges.

Chinese Braised Beef

The perfect dinner when you fancy something hearty and warming. It comes with some exotic flavours as well that are sure to intrigue you.

Serves 4

1 kg braising beef, cut into chunks
5 spring onions, finely diced
1 red chilli pepper, finely diced
300ml beef stock
125ml red wine
2 tbsp olive oil
2 cloves of garlic, finely diced
2.5cm root ginger, grated
2 tbsp plain flour
1 tsp Chinese five-spice powder
2 tbsp soy sauce

Preheat the oven to 160°C, gas mark 3.

Heat the olive oil in a large frying pan and fry the garlic, ginger, onions and chilli until cooked. Put them on a plate and place to one side.

Toss the beef in the flour then put it in the frying pan in batches as necessary. Cook each batch for about 5 minutes until brown.

Add the five-spice powder to the pan together with

cont'd

the onion, garlic, ginger and chilli mixture, and fry it for 2 minutes or so. Lastly, splash in the wine.

Transfer everything to a casserole dish and add the soy sauce and beef stock. Put the cover on the casserole dish and place it in the preheated oven.

Cook for 2 hours stirring the meat halfway through. The meat should be very soft, and any sinewy bits should have melted. It will now be ready to eat.

Chilli Con Carne

Originating from the American state of Texas, this dish consists of minced beef and beans smothered in a spicy chilli tomato sauce.

<u>Serves 4</u>

500g lean beef mince
1 onion, finely chopped
1 x 400g tin chopped tomatoes
1 x 400g tin haricot beans
2 garlic cloves, finely chopped
2 tbsp tomato puree
2 tsp ground cumin
1/2 tsp ground cinnamon
1 tsp dried chilli flakes
1 tsp paprika
1 tbsp olive oil

Fry the mince in the olive oil over a medium heat until it is browned, stirring often. Then add the onions and fry for another 5 minutes or so.

Add the remaining ingredients, stir well and bring to a simmer leaving it to cook until it has thickened.

Serve on a bed of mixed vegetables or rice. If you do use rice, go for brown, which is healthier.

Chicken & Chorizo Jambalaya

A Cajun-inspired rice pot recipe with spicy Spanish sausage, sweet peppers and tomatoes. Low-carb dry Shirataki rice is used instead of normal rice here.

<u>Serves 4</u>

2 chicken breasts, chopped
1 onion, chopped
1 bell pepper, thinly sliced
250g dry Shirataki rice
1 x 400g tin plum tomatoes
350ml chicken stock
2 garlic cloves, crushed
1 tbsp olive oil
75g chorizo, sliced
1 tbsp Cajun seasoning

Heat the oil in a large frying pan and fry the chicken until cooked through. Remove and put to one side.

Add the onion and cook for 5 minutes until it's brown. Then add the pepper, garlic, chorizo and Cajun seasoning, and cook for another 5 minutes.

Cook the Shirataki rice by simmering it in a pan of water for 20 minutes. Then drain the water and add the rice, the chicken and the chicken stock to the pan containing the pepper, garlic, chorizo and Cajun seasoning. Mix well and serve.

Simple Sauerkraut

This recipe is an easy way to make classic sauerkraut - a fermented food that provides enormous benefits for the digestive system.

Makes Approximately 4 Jars

2 kg green or white cabbage
3 tbsp rock salt
1 tsp caraway seeds
1 tsp peppercorns

Wash a large tub or bowl, then rinse it with boiling water. Make sure that your hands, and everything else coming into contact with the cabbage, are very clean.

Finely shred the cabbage – a food processor makes light work of this. Layer the cabbage and the salt in the tub/bowl. Rub the salt into the cabbage for 5 minutes, wait 5 minutes, then repeat. You should end up with a much reduced volume of cabbage sitting in its own brine. Then add the caraway seeds and the peppercorns.

Cover the surface of the cabbage with a sheet of cling film, then press out all the air bubbles. Weigh the cabbage down using a couple of heavy plates, or other weights that fit your tub/bowl, so that the level of the brine rises to cover the cabbage. Cover the tub/bowl with a lid, or cling film, and leave it in a dark place

cont'd

at a room temperature of about 20°C for at least 5 days.

When 5 days is up it will be ready to eat. However, for maximum flavour leave the cabbage to ferment for up to 6 weeks.

Check it every day, releasing any gases that have built up as it ferments, and give it a stir to release the bubbles. If any scum forms, remove it, rinse the weights in boiling water and replace the cling film. You should see bubbles appearing within the cabbage, and possibly some foam on the top of the brine.

It's important to keep it at a cool and even room temperature – too cool and the ferment will take longer than necessary. If it's too warm, the sauerkraut may become mouldy or ferment too quickly, leading to a less than perfect result.

The cabbage will become increasingly sour the longer it's fermented, so taste it now and again. When you are happy with it, transfer it to sterilised jars and put them in the fridge where the sauerkraut will keep for up to 6 months.

Spicy Nut Roast

An extremely satiating vegetarian loaf packed with nuts, fruit, spices and vegetables that is just perfect for an evening meal.

Serves 4

100g butternut squash, cut into chunks
1 onion, chopped
1 bell pepper, chopped
150g mixed unsalted nuts
150g ground almonds
200g cooked chestnuts, diced
2 eggs
250g spinach, chopped
25g dried cranberries
2 tbsp olive oil
2 cloves garlic, crushed
2 tbsp water
1 tsp ground nutmeg

Heat 1 tbsp of olive oil in a pan and cook the spinach, a handful at a time. As each handful wilts, add another. Cook for 2 or 3 minutes, stirring the spinach constantly. When done, put it to one side.

Place the butternut chunks in a pan of boiling water and boil until tender. Then mash them and put to one side as well.

cont'd

Next, heat the remaining olive oil in a pan, add the onion, pepper and garlic, and cook for about 5 minutes. Remove from the heat and allow to cool.

Divide the nuts into 3 piles. Put one aside, roughly chop the second pile and finely chop the third pile.

Put the eggs in a bowl together with the ground almonds, the cooked onion, pepper and garlic, finely chopped and roughly chopped nuts, the chestnuts, water and nutmeg. Mix thoroughly.

Line a 1 lb loaf tin with greaseproof paper. Then take two-thirds of the egg mixture and press it around the sides and bottom of the tin, leaving room in the middle for the filling.

Put the mashed butternut squash in the middle and layer the spinach on top. Sprinkle the cranberries on top of the spinach. Now add the rest of the egg mixture to create a lid and sprinkle it with the whole nuts, pressing them gently into the topping.

Cover the tin with a piece of foil and place it in a larger oven-proof dish. Fill the dish with enough water so that the lower half of the loaf tin is covered.

Cook the nut roast in the oven for 30 minutes at 170°C, then remove the foil and cook it for another 10 minutes. It will then be ready to eat.

Fish Stew

A hearty Mediterranean seafood dinner, packed with vegetables and garlic.

<u>Serves 4</u>

4 fish fillets, cut in half to give 8 pieces
150g king prawns
150g mussel meat
2 tomatoes, finely chopped
1 carrot, diced
1 bell pepper, sliced
1 leek, chopped
1 fish stock cube in 600ml of water
1/2 bulb fennel, sliced
1 tsp turmeric
2 cloves garlic, crushed
2 tbsp olive oil
1 tbsp finely chopped parsley

Put the water in a pan with the stock cube, bring to the boil, then turn down the heat. Cover and simmer for 5 minutes. Then add the carrot, fennel, pepper, leek, turmeric and garlic. Mix thoroughly, then cover and simmer for a further 5 minutes.

Next, put 1 tbsp of olive oil in a frying pan over a medium heat. When the pan is hot, add 4 pieces of fish and cook for 2-3 minutes. Turn them over and cook for another 1-2 minutes. Remove them from the

cont'd

pan and cook the other 4 pieces of fish with the second tablespoon of olive oil.

Add the mussels and prawns to the vegetables and stock, bring to the boil and cook for 2 minutes.

Put the vegetables, prawns, mussels and stock in four bowls. Place the fish fillets on top, sprinkle with parsley, chopped tomato and a sprinkle of black pepper. Serve.

Pumpkin Curry

A vegetarian dish very popular in Mediterranean countries where it is eaten as both dinner and lunch.

Serves 4

1 kg piece of pumpkin
2 onions, finely chopped
1 x 400ml tin coconut milk
1 x 400g tin chickpeas, drained and rinsed
3 stalks lemongrass
1 tbsp sesame oil
3 tbsp Thai yellow curry paste
8 cardamom pods
1 tbsp mustard seed
250ml vegetable stock
2 limes

Heat the sesame oil in a pan, then fry the curry paste with the onions, lemon-grass, cardamom pods and mustard seed for 4-5 minutes.

Stir the pumpkin into the pan and coat in the paste, then pour in the stock and coconut milk. Bring everything to a simmer, add the chickpeas, then cook for about 10 minutes until the pumpkin is tender.

Squeeze the juice of one lime into the curry, then cut the other lime into wedges to serve alongside.

Garlic Roasted Broccoli

With just a handful of ingredients, this dish is quick to make, tasty and very nutritious.

2 heads of broccoli, cut into florets
3 tbsp coconut oil
5 garlic cloves, finely chopped
1 lemon, juice of
Pinch of chilli flakes
Salt and pepper

Preheat the oven to 180°C, gas mark 4.

Melt the coconut oil in a small pan and then pour it into a bowl. Add the broccoli, salt, pepper and garlic and toss together until everything is coated in the coconut oil.

Lightly grease a baking tray and spread the broccoli mixture out in a layer. Place the tray in the preheated oven and bake until the broccoli florets are tender enough to pierce with a fork and the edges are beginning to turn brown. Turn once halfway through the baking process and add the chilli flakes.

After baking, squeeze the lemon juice liberally over the broccoli before serving.

Salmon Fish Cakes

If you're after something that's lighter than potato-packed fish cakes, try this oriental-style version.

4 salmon fillets, cut into chunks
2 carrots, cut into strips
1 small cucumber, cut into strips
2.5cm root ginger, grated
2 tbsp Thai red curry paste
1 tsp soy sauce
1 tbsp olive oil
1 lemon, cut into wedges
2 tbsp white wine vinegar
1 tsp caster sugar

Using a food processor, pulse the salmon, curry paste, ginger and soy sauce until roughly minced. Remove the mixture and shape it into four burger-size patties.

Heat the olive oil in a frying pan then fry the patties for 4-5 minutes on each side.

Next, put the strips of carrot and cucumber into a bowl. Add the sugar and vinegar, and toss until the sugar has dissolved.

Divide the salad between four plates with a fish cake on each plate. Serve with the lemon wedges.

Salad Recipes

Thai Chicken Salad

The hot spiciness of this salad works well with the vegetables, creating a good balance of flavour and heat.

4 chicken breasts, finely chopped
1 cucumber, cut into strips
200g bean sprouts
2 red chilli peppers
3 baby gem lettuces, leaves separated
3 cloves of garlic
2.5cm root ginger
1 tbsp sesame oil
1 tsp chilli powder
50ml fish sauce
3 tbsp lime juice

Blitz the chillies, garlic and ginger in a food processor.

Heat the sesame oil in a frying pan and then add the chilli and garlic mixture. Stir-fry for 1 minute and then add the chicken and chilli powder. Stir-fry for 4 minutes more before adding the fish sauce. Cook for another 5 minutes.

Remove from the heat and pour the lime juice over the chicken. Serve with the lettuce, cucumber and bean sprouts.

Asparagus & Egg Salad

A simple, balanced bistro-style salad that's low in calories but high in flavour, texture and nutrition.

<u>Serves 2</u>

200g beetroot, chopped
1/4 cucumber, cut into strips
8 asparagus spears, trimmed
2 eggs
1 tbsp olive oil
1 tbsp balsamic vinegar
Handful lettuce leaves

Put the beetroot in a saucepan, cover with water and bring it to the boil. Then reduce the heat to medium-low, cover and simmer for 40 minutes until it's tender.

Mix the olive oil and vinegar in a bowl and then add the cooked beetroot and toss to coat it.

Blanch the asparagus in a pan of hot water for 2 minutes, then remove and set aside. Crack the eggs into the pan and simmer until the whites are cooked and the yolks are just beginning to set. Remove and put to one side.

Now put the beetroot, lettuce and cucumber on 2 plates. Pour the olive oil and vinegar dressing over it and then top with the asparagus and a poached egg.

Squid & Pepper Salad

Found in every ocean, squid is one of the most widely available seafoods in the world, and is also one of the cheapest.

4 bell peppers, thinly sliced
600g squid, sliced into rings
2 x 400g tins chickpeas, rinsed and drained
1 red chilli pepper, chopped
2 garlic cloves, grated
4 tbsp olive oil
1 lemon, zest and juice of
Bunch of parsley, roughly chopped
Salt and pepper

Cook the peppers under the grill. Then put them in a large bowl together with the chickpeas, parsley, chilli and garlic. Mix thoroughly and put to one side.

Heat one tablespoon of olive oil in a frying pan and add the squid. Stir-fry it until cooked.

Then put the squid into the bowl that contains the peppers and other ingredients. Season everything with salt and pepper and then dress with the remaining oil, lemon juice and lemon zest.

Serve.

Lemon & Feta Salad

A fresh and tasty salad that could have been designed for a summer's day. The pine nuts give it a deliciously crunchy texture.

<u>Serves 4</u>

250g spinach
1 tbsp pine nuts
30g feta cheese
1 lemon, zest and juice of
1 tbsp olive oil
Black pepper

Place the spinach in a pan of boiling water. Let it cook for 3-5 minutes and then remove it from the pan. Put to one side.

Roast the pine nuts in a dry pan for a couple of minutes, stirring constantly until they are just starting to brown.

Spread the spinach on a plate and crumble the feta cheese over it. Scatter the roasted pine nuts on top.

Finish by sprinkling the lemon zest over the dish and drizzling it with the lemon juice and olive oil.

Season with the black pepper and serve.

Falafel Tabbouleh Salad

A platter salad that's perfect for the whole family to share.

Serves 4

16 ready-made falafels
200g couscous
5 spring onions, finely sliced
1 cucumber, sliced
2 lemons, zest and juice of
150ml yoghurt
3 tbsp olive oil
Small bunch mint leaves, chopped
Small bunch parsley leaves, chopped

Cook the falafels according to the pack instructions.

Put the couscous into a bowl with 350ml of boiling water, mix, then leave until all the water is absorbed.

Fluff the couscous with a fork, then add the lemon zest, half the lemon juice, olive oil, spring onions, cucumber, mint and three-quarters of the parsley. Mix thoroughly and then put it on a platter.

Mix the remaining lemon juice and parsley into the yoghurt, then put the mixture into a bowl.

Scatter the hot falafels over the couscous salad on the platter and serve with the yoghurt sauce.

Probiotic Cabbage Salad

This salad is full of digestion-supportive enzymes and probiotics that provide incredible health benefits.

750g red cabbage, finely shredded
75g tahini paste
1 tbsp apple cider vinegar
1 tsp himalayan rock salt
50g nutritional yeast flakes
2 tsp coconut nectar
Cayenne pepper, to taste
1 capsule raw probiotics

Dressing:
Handful of parsley, chopped
Handful of alfalfa sprouts
Dash of cayenne pepper

Mix the cabbage, tahini, vinegar, salt, yeast flakes, coconut nectar and pepper together in a large salad bowl.

Open the probiotic capsule and pour the contents into the bowl as well. Put the bowl to one side.

Now prepare the dressing by mixing the parsley, alfalfa sprouts and pepper in another bowl.

Top the salad with the dressing and serve.

Fire Salad

Fajita seasoning makes this chicken salad a seriously HOT affair! It's also seriously high in nutrients.

Serves 4

2 chicken breast fillets
1 x 35g packet of Old El Paso Fajita Spice Mix
1 x 400g tin black beans, rinsed and drained
1 onion, chopped
1 tomato, chopped
300g sweetcorn
300g mixed salad greens
100g salsa sauce
1 tbsp olive oil

Coat the chicken with half of the fajita spice mix. Then heat the olive oil in a frying pan and cook the chicken for 8 minutes on each side. Cut it into strips and put them to one side.

In a saucepan, mix the beans, sweetcorn, salsa sauce and the other half of the fajita seasoning. Heat over a medium heat until warm.

Then mix the salad greens, onion and tomato in a bowl and top with the chicken. Finally, dress it all with the bean and corn mixture.

Avocado Salad

A favourite summer salad! The pumpkin seeds add texture and are also very nutritious.

<u>Serves 4</u>

2 heads little gem lettuce
2 avocados - de-stoned and sliced
50g pumpkin seeds
1 tbsp red wine vinegar
1 tbsp balsamic vinegar
1 clove garlic, diced
1 tbsp mayonnaise
6 tbsp olive oil
1 lime, juice of
Salt and pepper

Whisk the olive oil, lime juice, red wine vinegar, balsamic vinegar, garlic and mayonnaise together to make the dressing.

Season the dressing with salt and pepper to taste.

Put the lettuce and pumpkin seeds in a salad bowl and mix them. Toss with enough dressing to coat the salad thoroughly.

Top with the sliced avocado and serve.

Probiotic Green Salad

This salad contains natural probiotics which helps clean the intestines, thus improving the efficiency with which nutrients can be absorbed.

<u>Serves 4</u>

1 white or red cabbage
2 carrots
5cm root ginger
1 tbsp miso paste
350ml water
1/2 tsp cayenne powder

Shred the cabbage, carrots and ginger, either by hand or in a food processor.

In a bowl, mix the miso paste, water and cayenne powder. Then, in a large bowl, toss the shredded cabbage, carrots and ginger with the blended miso paste, water and cayenne powder.

Pack the mixture as tightly as you can in a mason jar. It is very important to do this as tight packing eliminates as much air as possible.

Close the jar tightly and let it stand outside. The salad can be eaten immediately but as the days go by it will ferment. When it does, the good bacteria will flourish, giving the salad its detoxification properties.

Red Cabbage & Kale Salad

Crunchy red cabbage, crisp kale, spicy chilli flakes and juicy pomegranate seeds make a salad is that is packed with colour and flavour.

<u>Serves 4</u>

1/2 red cabbage, finely chopped
1 onion, chopped
100g kale, chopped
80g pomegranate seeds
2 garlic cloves, chopped
1/2 tsp crushed chilli
2 tbsp olive oil

Dressing:
2 tbsp tahini
2 tbsp yoghurt
1/2 lemon, juice of

Heat the oil in a frying pan. Add the onion and cook until it's nicely browned. Remove and put to one side.

Put the cabbage and kale in the same pan and cook for 8 minutes. Stir in the garlic and chilli and cook for a further 2 minutes. Transfer to a bowl and toss with the onion and pomegranate seeds.

Mix all the dressing ingredients in a bowl with 1 tbsp of water. Drizzle over the salad and serve.

Indian Summer Salad

Packed with antioxidants, this super-healthy, colourful salad counts as one of your 5-a-day.

3 carrots
5 radishes
2 courgettes
1 onion
Handful mint leaves, chopped
1 tbsp white wine vinegar
1 tsp Dijon mustard
1 tbsp mayonnaise
2 tbsp olive oil
Salt and pepper

Grate the three carrots into a bowl. Then thinly slice the radishes and courgettes and finely chop the onion. Mix all the vegetables together in the bowl with the mint leaves.

Make the dressing by putting the vinegar, mustard and mayonnaise in a bowl and whisking to a smooth creamy consistency. Then gradually whisk in the olive oil.

Add salt and pepper to taste and then drizzle the dressing over the salad before serving.

Soup Recipes

Chickpea Soup

Come home to a bowl of this filling, low-fat soup. It's perfect for vegetarians as well.

Serves 4

1 x 400g tin chopped tomatoes
1 x 400g tin chickpeas, rinsed and drained
100g broad beans
1 onion, chopped
2 celery sticks, chopped
2 tsp ground cumin
500ml vegetable stock
1/2 lemon, zest and juice of
1 handful coriander or parsley, chopped
1 tbsp olive oil
Pinch of black pepper

Heat the oil in a large saucepan, then fry the onion and celery until softened, stirring frequently. Add the cumin and fry for another minute.

Add the vegetable stock, tomatoes and chickpeas, plus a good pinch of black pepper. Simmer for 8 minutes and then add the broad beans and lemon juice. Cook for a further 2 minutes.

Season to taste, top with a sprinkling of lemon zest and chopped coriander or parsley, and serve.

Kale & Chicken Soup

This soup has tender chicken, savoury broth and grain-free noodles.

1 onion, finely chopped
500ml chicken stock
1 chicken breast
150g kale, finely chopped
225g egg noodles
2 garlic cloves, diced
1/2 tsp fennel seed
1 tsp salt
3 tbsp olive oil
1 lemon, zest of
Handful of rosemary, chopped

Start by cooking the noodles. To do this, place them in a large pan and cover with boiling water. Leave them to boil until soft enough to eat (or follow the timing instructions on the packaging).

Heat the olive oil in a large pan, then add the onion, garlic, fennel seed, rosemary and salt. Cook for about 5 minutes over a medium heat until the onions are browned.

Then add the stock and bring to a simmer. Next, add the chicken breast, cover the pot and leave the chicken

cont'd

to cook for 15 minutes.

When it's ready, remove it from the pot and place it on one side to cool.

When it has cooled sufficiently to handle, shred it as finely as you can. Add it and the kale to the soup pot and bring to a simmer. It will now be ready to eat.

To serve, ladle the soup over the cooked noodles and finish with a sprinkle of salt and the lemon zest.

Bulgar Mushroom Soup

This soup from Eastern Europe is primarily a mushroom soup but it gets a lot of extra flavour from the other ingredients.

1 onion, chopped
2 large mushrooms, chopped
250ml milk
3 tbsp plain flour
500ml chicken stock
125ml sour cream
50g butter
2 tsp dried dill
1 tbsp paprika
1 tbsp soy sauce
2 tsp lemon juice
Handful chopped parsley
Salt and pepper

Melt the butter in a large pot over a medium heat, add the onions and cook them until brown.

Add the mushrooms and cook for 5 more minutes.

Stir in the dill, paprika, soy sauce and chicken stock. Then reduce the heat to low, cover the pot and leave it to simmer for 15 minutes.

cont'd

In a bowl, whisk the milk and flour together and then pour the mix into the soup. Stir well, cover and simmer for another 15 minutes.

Finally, add the salt, pepper, lemon juice, parsley and sour cream. Mix thoroughly, heat up for a couple of minutes and then serve.

Oriental Pumpkin Soup

Flavours of the mysterious East give this seasonal soup an added twist.

750g pumpkin, finely chopped
1 onion, sliced
1 red chilli pepper, sliced
500ml vegetable stock
200ml coconut milk
1 tbsp ginger, grated
3 tbsp Thai red curry paste
2 tbsp olive oil
1 tsp lime juice
1 tsp sugar

Put the pumpkin in a roasting tin and mix it with 1 tbsp of olive oil, half the lime juice and the sugar. Roast it for 30 minutes in an oven set at 200°C.

In a pan, fry the onion and ginger in the remaining olive oil for about 5 minutes until soft. Then add the curry paste, the roasted pumpkin, all but 3 tbsp of the coconut milk and the stock. Bring to a simmer and leave it for 5 minutes.

Now whisk the soup with a blender until it is smooth. Add the remaining lime juice and serve drizzled with the remaining coconut milk and the chilli slices.

Ginger & Carrot Soup

This soup gets its probiotics from miso, a Japanese paste made by fermenting soybeans. It adds a rich, savoury flavour to dishes.

Serves 4

1 onion, chopped
600ml vegetable stock
5 carrots, chopped
200ml coconut milk
5cm root ginger, grated
2 tbsp coconut oil
2 tsp tamari (or soy sauce)
3 tbsp miso paste
2 tbsp sesame seeds, crushed

Melt the coconut oil in a large pot over a medium heat. Add the onions and cook until browned. Then add the vegetable stock, carrots, ginger and tamari. Bring to a boil, then reduce the heat and let the soup simmer for about 5 minutes until the carrots have softened.

After about 10 minutes when the soup has cooled, put it in a food processor together with the coconut milk and miso paste. Blend until smooth and creamy.

Scatter the crushed sesame seeds over the top, add salt and pepper to taste and then serve.

Prawn & Mushroom Soup

A quick and spicy wok-based soup means one pan, zero fuss and supper on the table in just a few minutes.

<u>Serves 4</u>

300g bag of stir-fry vegetables
150g shiitake mushrooms, sliced
1 x 400g tin coconut milk
200ml fish stock
300g noodles
200g prawns
2 tbsp Thai green curry paste
2 sprigs parsley, chopped
1 tbsp olive oil

Heat the olive oil in the wok, then add and stir-fry the vegetables and the mushrooms for 2-3 minutes. Remove them from the wok and put to one side.

Put the curry paste into the wok and fry for 1 min.

Pour in the coconut milk and fish stock. Bring to the boil, drop in the noodles and prawns, then reduce the heat and simmer for 4 minutes until the prawns are cooked through. Stir in the vegetables, mushrooms and the chopped parsley.

The soup is now ready to serve.

Peanut Soup

A hearty soup which gets its delicious flavour and enticing colour from a combination of red peppers, tomatoes, peanut butter, chilli pepper and brown rice.

Serves 4

1 onion, chopped
1 red pepper, chopped
700g jar passata
1 ltr vegetable stock
200g crunchy peanut butter
85g uncooked brown rice
2 cloves garlic, minced
1/2 tsp black pepper
1/2 tsp chilli powder
2 tbsp olive oil

Heat the oil in a large saucepan over a medium heat. Cook the onions and pepper until tender. Stir in the garlic when nearly done.

Add the passata, vegetable stock, black pepper and chilli powder. Reduce the heat to low and simmer, uncovered, for 20 minutes.

Add the rice, cover the pan, and simmer for another 40 minutes until the rice is tender. Finally, stir in the peanut butter until it is well blended. Serve.

Beet & Garlic Soup

This super gut-friendly soup has three sources of prebiotics - leeks, garlic, and beets.

<u>Serves 4</u>

4 beetroots
2 leeks, sliced
1 ltr vegetable stock
2 heads garlic
4 tbsp avocado oil
2 tsp lemon juice
Salt and pepper to taste

Pre-heat the oven to 190°C, gas mark 5.

Drizzle the beetroots with 1 tbsp of avocado oil and then wrap them tightly in parchment lined foil. Cut the tops off the garlic heads (leaving the bulbs intact), and drizzle them with 1 tbsp of avocado oil as well. As with the beets, wrap them tightly in parchment lined foil. Place the wrapped beets and garlic heads on a baking tray and place it in the oven.

Roast the beets and garlic heads for 45 minutes, then remove them from the oven and allow to cool. Peel and chop the beets into chunks. Split the garlic heads into individual cloves, peel them and then chop them finely.

In a large pot, heat the remaining 2 tbsp of avocado

cont'd

oil over a medium heat. Add the leeks and cook them until they are just brown. Add the chopped and roasted garlic and beets, then top with the vegetable stock. Bring to the boil.

Turn off the heat, cover the pot and let it sit for ten minutes before pouring it into a food processor. Add the lemon juice and blend until the soup is smooth and creamy.

Season with salt and pepper and serve.

Summer Miso Soup

Miso soup is deliciously savoury and comforting. And, with a good quality stock, it is a dish that takes only a few minutes to prepare.

<u>Serves 4</u>

20g instant dashi (Japanese stock)
200g silken tofu
800ml boiling water
4 asparagus spears
2 tbsp miso paste
1 tbsp mirin (sweet rice wine)
1 tbsp soy sauce

Mix the dashi with the boiling water in a saucepan and stir well.

Finely slice the asparagus spears and add them to the pan. Simmer for three minutes.

Put the miso paste and silken tofu in a small bowl and add a ladleful of the hot broth, whisking to get rid of any lumps. When it's smooth, pour the mixture back into the saucepan.

Add the mirin and soy sauce. Heat and then serve.

Radish Noodle Soup

This daikon noodle soup is gluten-free and quick and easy to make. Daikon radish is very good for digestion, and for the immune system particularly.

Serves 4

1 large daikon radish
1 chilli pepper, finely chopped
1 tbsp raw apple cider vinegar
1 tbsp dill, chopped
2 garlic cloves, crushed
Pinch of rock salt

Peel the daikon radish and, using a spiralizer, make it into noodles. Then place the noodles into a mason jar and add the chopped chilli peppers, apple cider vinegar, dill, garlic and salt.

Pour spring water all the way to the mouth of the jar (so there is as little air as possible) and seal tightly.

Place the mason jar in a dark, warm place and let the soup ferment for 2 or 3 days. Then refrigerate.

Simply warm it up when you are ready to eat it.

Snack Recipes

Chargrilled Corn on the Cob

Bring your barbeque to life with these colourful corn on the cobs. Sweet, succulent and an excellent way to get your five-a-day.

<u>**Serves 4**</u>

4 cobs of corn
Salt and pepper

Dip:
225g fromage frais
2 spring onions, chopped
1 tbsp chives, chopped
1 tbsp mint, chopped
1 red chilli pepper, finely chopped
1/2 lemon, juice of

Cut each cob in half. Parboil them in a large saucepan of boiling water for about 5 minutes until tender. Then remove them from the pan and pat dry with kitchen paper.

Spray the cobs with cooking spray and place them under a heated grill or over a barbecue. Grill for 2 to 3 minutes, turning frequently, until slightly charred.

Meanwhile, mix the ingredients for the herb dip and put it in a serving bowl. Season the cooked corn cobs with salt and pepper and serve with the dip.

Quinoa Muffins

High in protein, these savoury muffins with quinoa and feta cheese can be eaten either hot or cold.

Makes 8

250g quinoa, cooked
100g almonds, ground
1 onion, chopped
3 eggs
50g feta cheese
50g kale, finely chopped
1 tbsp olive oil
1 clove of garlic, crushed

Preheat the oven to 180°C, gas mark 4.

Line a muffin tray with paper muffin cases and grease them lightly with olive oil.

Beat the eggs in a bowl. Then add the onion, garlic, kale, quinoa and ground almonds. Crumble in the feta cheese, mix thoroughly and season to taste.

Spoon the mixture into the muffin cases and bake for 20-25 minutes or until golden brown.

Remove the muffins from the oven and serve.

Granola Bars

These blueberry and yoghurt granola bars can be eaten for breakfast, as a snack or for dessert.

<u>**Makes 10 bars**</u>

300g rolled oats
225g brown rice krispies
75g almonds, chopped
75g almond butter
75g honey
75g blueberries
50g shredded coconut
1 tbsp chia seeds
2 tsp vanilla extract

Greek Yoghurt Coating:
50g Greek yoghurt
1 tbsp honey
1 tbsp water
1 tsp vanilla extract
1/2 tsp gelatin

In a large bowl, mix the oats, rice krispies, coconut, almonds and chia seeds. Then, in a separate bowl, mix the almond butter and honey. Microwave the latter for 30 seconds to 1 minute. Add the vanilla extract and mix again.

Add the honey, almond and vanilla mixture to the oat

cont'd

mixture and mix well before adding the blueberries. Put the mixture into a dish, packing it in tightly and put it in the freezer. When it has frozen, remove it from the freezer, cut it into ten bars and then put the bars back in the freezer.

Next, make the Greek yoghurt coating. Mix the water and vanilla in a small bowl. Sprinkle the gelatin over the top and whisk until it has set into a thick paste. Put it to one side.

In another small bowl mix the yoghurt and honey and microwave it for 30 seconds. Then add the gelatin mixture to it and whisk until it has dissolved.

Dip the bottom of the bars into the yoghurt coating and let the excess drip off before placing them on a plate. When the yoghurt is dry, coat the top of the bars.

Wait for the tops to dry and they will then be ready to eat.

Lemon Houmous

Houmous is so easy to make and beats shop-bought versions every time.

2 x 400g tins chickpeas, drained
2 garlic cloves, finely chopped
3 tbsp yoghurt
3 tbsp Tahini paste
3 tbsp olive oil
2 lemons, zest and juice of
1 tsp coriander
Salt and pepper

Put the chickpeas, garlic cloves, yoghurt, Tahini paste, lemon zest and lemon juice into a food processor. Whisk the ingredients to a smooth consistency.

Remove the houmous mixture from the processor and put it in a bowl. Season it with salt and pepper and then scatter the coriander on top.

Drizzle with olive oil and serve.

Squash Chunks

Chunky wedges of squash covered in a crispy, spicy coating of nuts and seeds. Extremely nutritious.

<u>Serves 4</u>

1 butternut squash
50g hazelnuts
1 tbsp coriander seeds
2 tbsp sesame seeds
1 tbsp ground cumin
1 tbsp olive oil

Preheat the oven to 200°C, gas mark 6.

Toast the hazelnuts in a frying pan over a medium heat until golden. Add the coriander and sesame seeds, and toast for 1 more minute. Set aside. When cool, place in a blender together with the ground cumin and whisk until thoroughly mixed.

Peel the butternut squash, remove the seeds and slice it into chunks. Toss the chunks with the olive oil, then cover them with the nut and seed coating.

Line a baking tray with greaseproof paper and add the coated chunks in a single layer. Cook for 30-40 minutes, turning halfway through, until tender.

Berry Kombucha Biscuits

This delicious and unusual snack is made with fresh berries, kombucha and agave syrup - ingredients that are all very good for your digestive system.

Serves 2

225g mixed berries, chopped
150g berry flavoured kombucha
4 tbsp gelatin
2 tbsp agave syrup

Put the mixed berries in a food processor and puree the berries. Then sieve the puree into a large bowl to remove the seeds.

In a small pot over a very low heat, warm the kombucha for about 1-2 minutes. Gradually whisk in the gelatin until it has dissolved.

Now add the pureed berries and agave syrup, and whisk until they are well combined.

Pour the mixture into biscuit moulds and leave to harden.

The kombucha biscuits are then ready to eat.

Chicken Satay Pieces

Keep these nutty chicken satay strips in the fridge for a healthy option when you're feeling a bit peckish.

Serves 2

2 chicken breast fillets cut into thick strips
2 tbsp chunky peanut butter
1 garlic clove, finely grated
1 tsp Madras curry powder
1 tbsp soy sauce
2 tsp lime juice
Sweet chilli sauce

Preheat the oven to 200°C, gas mark 6.

Put the peanut butter, garlic, curry powder, soy sauce and lime juice in a bowl and mix well. If necessary, add a splash of boiling water to achieve the thickish consistency necessary for coating.

Add the chicken strips to the bowl and mix thoroughly ensuring they are well coated. Then place the strips in a baking tin lined with greaseproof paper and cook in the oven for about 10 minutes.

Eat with the chilli sauce.

Sourdough Oat Bran Muffins

These sourdough muffins are full of low-glycemic bran that your digestive system will just love.

Makes 12 Muffins

300g sourdough starter
225g wheat or oat bran
100g flour
3 tbsp melted butter
3 tbsp honey
3 tbsp raisins
2 eggs
2 tsp cinnamon
2 tsp baking soda
1/2 tsp nutmeg, grated

Preheat the oven to 220°C, gas mark 7.

Mix the starter, bran and flour in a bowl. Cover and place in a warm spot to ferment for 8 to 12 hours.

In a bowl, whisk together the eggs, butter, honey, nutmeg and cinnamon.

Sprinkle the baking soda over the fermented dough and gradually stir it in along with the egg mixture and raisins.

Divide the batter into 12 muffin cups and bake in the preheated oven for about 15 minutes.

Stuffed Mushrooms

Mushrooms stuffed with blue cheese, bacon, onions and garlic make a delicious and very nutritious snack.

4 strips bacon
4 large mushrooms
1 onion, diced
100g cream cheese
100g blue cheese
1 tbsp butter
1 tsp olive oil

Preheat the oven to 175°C, gas mark 4.

Fry the bacon in the olive oil and put it to one side. Remove the stems from the mushrooms and chop them up. Put the caps to one side.

Put the butter in a pan with the mushroom stems and onion. Cook them for about 7 minutes.

Then put the onion and mushroom mixture into a food processor together with the bacon, cream cheese and blue cheese. Blend to a smooth consistency.

Stuff the mixture into the mushroom caps and put them in a baking tin lined with greaseproof paper. Bake in the oven for 15 minutes.

Salmon Mayonnaise Wraps

Packed with omega-3-rich salmon, these delicious wraps with avocado and mayonnaise are an extremely healthy low-carb, high-protein snack.

Serves 2

2 salmon fillets
8 lettuce leaves
1 avocado
16 cherry tomatoes, halved
1/2 tsp mustard powder
1 tbsp capers
1 tsp cider vinegar
1 tsp olive oil

Brush the salmon fillets with the olive oil, put them into a pan and cook for 3-4 minutes on each side.

Scoop the avocado's meat into a bowl. Add the mustard powder and vinegar, then mash well so that the mixture has a smooth mayonnaise-like consistency. Stir in the capers. Spoon into two small dishes and put on serving plates with the lettuce leaves and tomatoes.

Slice the salmon and arrange on the plates. Spoon some of the 'mayonnaise' onto the lettuce leaves and top with salmon and cherry tomatoes. To eat, roll the lettuce leaves into wraps.

Dessert Recipes

Chocolate Kefir Ice Cream

If you avoid ice cream thinking it's unhealthy, give this one a try. It contains kefir - a cultured, probiotic yoghurt-like product that is rich in vitamins and minerals, and contains easily digestible proteins.

Makes 1.5 Litres

500ml coconut milk or cream
500ml full cream milk
75g cocoa powder
1 avocado
3 egg yolks
100g dates, chopped
25g plain kefir
2 tbsp vanilla extract

Place all the ingredients in a food processor and blitz until smooth and creamy.

Chill thoroughly before placing the ice cream in the freezer.

Allow it to harden for at least 1 hour before serving.

Coconut Macaroons

These easy-to-make macaroons are a very light yet satisfying dessert.

Serves 2

4 egg whites
250g desiccated coconut
75g dark chocolate
3 tbsp honey
1 tbsp coconut oil
2 tsp vanilla extract
1 pinch of salt

Preheat the oven to 160°C, gas mark 3.

Whisk the egg whites with the salt until stiff. Then add the honey, vanilla, desiccated coconut and coconut oil, and mix thoroughly.

Using a tablespoon, put large dollops of the macaroon mixture into a baking tin lined with greaseproof paper. Then bake for about 15 minutes until just starting to turn brown. Remove from the oven.

Finally, melt the dark chocolate and then drizzle it over the cooked macaroons.

Blueberry Muffins

These muffins are on a different level to the average muffin because they include probiotic-rich kefir.

Makes 12

300g whole wheat flour
200g blueberries
150g blueberry kefir
2 eggs
2 tbsp olive oil
1 tsp baking powder
1 tsp baking soda
1 tsp salt
1/2 tsp sugar
1 tsp vanilla

For the topping:
2 tbsp quick oats
2 tbsp brown sugar
1 tbsp butter

Preheat the oven to 200°C, gas mark 6.

Mix the flour, baking soda, baking powder and salt in a bowl and put to one side.

In another bowl, beat together the olive oil, eggs, sugar and vanilla.

cont'd

Now mix the contents of both bowls together thoroughly and then add the blueberry kefir to form the batter. If it is a bit dry, add a little more kefir. Finally, mix the blueberries into the batter.

Place paper cups in a muffin tray and scoop the batter into the cups.

Now mix the butter, sugar and oats and sprinkle a little of this on the top of each muffin.

Bake for about 20 minutes.

Berry Crumble

This scrumptious and super-healthy dessert is not only low in carbohydrates, it is sugar-free and gluten-free as well.

300g mixed berries
150g almonds
75g pecans
2 tbsp butter
1 tsp coconut oil
1 tsp cinnamon
1 tsp vanilla extract
1/4 tsp salt
5-10 drops liquid stevia sweetener (optional)

Preheat the oven to 200°C, gas mark 6.

Heat the coconut oil in a pan then add the berries and cook them for 3-5 minutes.

To make the crumble, put the almonds and pecans in a food processor. Add the butter, cinnamon, vanilla, salt and stevia (if using). Blitz for a few seconds until the mixture is chopped to a fine consistency.

Put the crumble in an oven-proof dish and sprinkle the berries on top. Cook for 10 minutes, remove from the oven and serve.

Lemon Squares

These lemon squares don't just taste delicious, they are also very good for you.

Serves 4

150g almond flour
4 eggs
2 tbsp butter, melted
2 tbsp lemon juice
1 tbsp coconut oil, melted
1 tbsp vanilla extract
1 tbsp honey
1/4 tsp salt

Preheat the oven to 175°C, gas mark 4.

To make the crust, put the almond flour, salt, coconut oil, butter and vanilla extract in a bowl and mix it all thoroughly into a dough.

Line a medium size baking tin with greaseproof paper and press the dough evenly into the bottom of the tin. Bake it for about 15 minutes until lightly brown.

While the crust is baking, prepare the topping. In a food processor, mix the almond flour, honey, eggs and lemon juice to a smooth consistency.

Remove the crust from the oven and pour the topping evenly all over it. Then return it to the oven and bake

cont'd

it for another 15 minutes until the topping is brown at the edges.

Remove from the oven and let it cool. Then put it in the refrigerator for 2 hours to allow it to set.

Cut into squares and serve.

Cacao & Coconut Pudding

This delicious pudding is literally brimming with healthy ingredients - protein, antioxidants, healthy fats and probiotics.

<u>Serves 2</u>

200g of shredded coconut
150g coconut milk
100g kefir
100g cacao nibs
100g collagen protein powder
1 tbsp honey
1 tsp vanilla extract

Soak the cacao nibs in water for 3 hours until they have softened. Then drain.

Next, put the softened nibs into a food processor, together with all the other ingredients. Blitz to a smooth and creamy consistency.

Remove the pudding mixture from the processor, place it in a bowl and refrigerate it for 1-2 hours.

Serve chilled.

Saffron Pannacotta

An enticing and extremely delicious dessert, this low-carb pannacotta is very easy to make.

Serves 2

12 raspberries
300g heavy whipping cream
1/2 tbsp gelatin powder
1 tbsp almonds, chopped
1/2 tsp vanilla extract
1/2 tsp saffron

Mix the gelatin powder with water (follow the instructions on the pack) and put to one side.

In a pan, boil the cream, vanilla and saffron. Reduce the heat and let it simmer for 10 minutes.

Remove the pan from the heat and add the gelatin. Stir until it has completely dissolved.

Pour the pannacotta mixture into 6 glasses. Cover the top of the glasses with plastic wrap and put them in the refrigerator for at least 2 hours.

Toast the almonds in a dry, hot, frying pan for a few minutes and then put them on top of the glasses of pannacotta, together with the raspberries.

Serve.

Chocolate & Peanut Squares

Chocolate and peanut butter could have been made for each other! The nuts give added crunchiness.

<u>Serves 2</u>

100g dark chocolate (cocoa content of at least 70%)
4 tbsp coconut oil
4 tbsp peanuts, finely chopped
4 tbsp peanut butter
1/2 tsp vanilla extract
1 tsp ground cinnamon
Pinch of salt

Melt the chocolate and coconut oil in a pan. Then add the salt, peanut butter, vanilla and cinnamon. Mix thoroughly to form a batter.

Pour the batter into a small baking tin lined with greaseproof paper.

Let it cool for a while and then top with the chopped peanuts. Refrigerate.

When the batter is set, cut it into small squares.

Store them in the refrigerator.

Pumpkin Pie

Sweet pumpkin, succulent coconut and a hint of lemon, all enveloped in a creamy filling. What could be nicer!

Serves 4

450g pumpkin, cut into chunks
100g heavy whipping cream
3 eggs
4 tbsp shredded coconut
2 tsp pumpkin pie spice
1 lemon, zest of
1 tbsp butter
1 tsp salt
1 tsp baking powder

Preheat the oven to 200°C, gas mark 6.

Put the pumpkin chunks in a pan. Add the whipping cream, butter and salt, and bring to the boil. Then reduce the heat and let it simmer for 20 minutes.

Next, put the pumpkin mixture, the pumpkin pie spice, coconut, eggs, lemon zest and baking powder, in a food processor and blitz to a smooth batter.

Pour the batter into an oven-proof dish and bake it for 20 minutes.

Then serve.

Nutritional Value of Fresh Fruit

	Calories	Fiber	Fat	Protein	Carbs
Apple - 1 medium	95	4.5g	0.5g	0.5g	25g
Apricot - 1 medium	14	0.5g	0g	0.5g	3g
Banana - 1 medium	105	3g	0.5g	1.5g	27g
Blackberry - 1 cup	62	7.5g	0.5g	2g	14g
Blueberry - 1 cup	83	3.5g	0.5g	1g	21g
Cherry - 1 cup	74	2.5g	0g	1g	19g
Coconut meat - 1 cup	283	7g	27g	2.5g	12g
Cranberry - 1 cup	60	4g	0g	0g	10g
Dates - 1 cup	495	15g	0g	4g	133g
Elderberry - 1 cup	106	10g	0.5g	1g	27g
Figs - 1 cup	492	20g	2g	6g	127g
Grapes - 1 cup	110	1g	0g	1g	27g
Grapefruit - 1 medium	82	3g	0g	1.5g	20g
Guava - 1 medium	61	5g	1g	2.5g	13g
Kiwi - 1 medium	42	2g	0.5g	1g	10g
Lemon - 1 medium	17	1.5g	0g	0.5g	5.5g
Lime - 1 medium	20	2g	0g	0.5g	7g
Mango - 1 medium	145	3.5g	0.5g	1g	35g
Mulberry - 1 cup	60	2.5g	0.5g	2g	14g
Orange - 1 medium	62	3g	0g	1g	15g
Papaya - 1 cup	60	2.5g	0.5g	0.5g	16g
Passion Fruit - 1 med	5	0.5g	0.5g	0.5g	1g
Peach - 1 medium	38	1.5g	0g	1g	9g
Pear - 1 medium	96	5g	0g	0.5g	25g
Plum - 1 medium	20	0.5g	0g	0.5g	5g
Pineapple - 1 cup	82	2.5g	0g	1g	21g
Pomegranate - 1 med	100	1g	0.5g	1g	26g
Raspberry - 1 cup	64	8g	1g	1.5g	15g
Rhubarb - 1 cup	26	2g	0g	1g	5.5g
Strawberry - 1 cup	49	3g	0.5g	1g	12g
Watermelon - 1 cup	45	0.5g	0g	1g	11g

Nutritional Value of Dried Fruit

	Calories	Fiber	Fat	Protein	Carbs
Apple - 1 cup	240	6g	0g	1g	50g
Apricots - 1 cup	310	9.5g	0.5g	4.5g	82g
Cranberries - 1 cup	520	8g	0g	0g	136g
Dates - 1 cup	493	15g	0g	4g	133g
Figs - 1 cup	490	20g	2g	6g	127g
Goji Berries - 1 cup	300	2g	3g	18g	60g
Prunes - 1 cup	408	12g	0.5g	3.5g	109g
Raisins - 1 cup	436	5g	1g	4g	115g
Sultanas - 1 cup	656	4.5g	0g	4.5g	154g

Nutritional Value of Dried Fruit

	Calories	Fiber	Fat	Protein	Carbs
Apple - 1 cup	117	0g	0.5g	0g	29g
Beetroot - 1 cup	96	0g	0g	3g	21g
Carrot - 1 cup	80	0g	0g	2g	17g
Cranberry - 1 cup	110	0g	0g	0g	28g
Grapefruit - 1 cup	96	0g	0g	1g	23g
Lemon - 1 tablespoon	3	0g	0g	0g	1g
Lime - 1 tablespoon	5	0g	0g	0g	1.5g
Orange - 1 cup	112	0.5g	0.5g	1.5g	26g
Pineapple - 1 cup	120	0g	0g	0g	31g
Pomegranate - 1 cup	100	0g	0g	0g	20g
Prune - 1cup	180	2.5g	0g	1.5g	45g
Tomato - 1 cup	41	1g	0g	2g	10g
Coconut water - 1 cup	46	2.5g	0.5g	1.5g	9g

Nutritional Value of Vegetables

	Calories	Fiber	Fat	Protein	Carbs
Artichoke - 1 medium	60	7g	0g	4g	13g
Asparagus - 1 cup	27	3g	0g	3g	5g
Avocado - 1 medium	289	12g	26.5g	3.5g	15g
Beetroot - 1 medium	35	2.5g	0g	1.5g	8g
Broccoli - 1 cup	31	2.5g	0.5g	2.5g	6g
Brussels Sprouts - 1 cup	38	3.5g	0.5g	3g	8g
Cabbage - 1 cup	22	2g	0g	1g	5g
Carrots - 1 medium	25	1.5g	0g	0.5g	6g
Cauliflower - 1 cup	25	2.5g	0g	2g	5.5g
Celery - 1 stalk	6	0.5g	0g	0.5g	1g
Courgette - 1 medium	40	2g	1g	3.5g	5g
Cucumber - 1 medium	24	1.5g	0.5g	1g	4.5g
Eggplant - 1 medium	21	3g	0.5g	1g	5g
Fennel - 1 medium	73	7g	0.5g	3g	17g
Ginger - 1 teaspoon	1.5	1g	0g	0g	1g
Green Beans - 1 cup	34	3.5g	0g	2g	8g
Kale - 1 cup	33	1g	1g	0.5g	7g
Lettuce - 1 cup	10	0g	0g	1g	2g
Mushrooms - 1 cup	15	1g	0g	2g	2g
Onion - 1 medium	47	2.5g	0g	1.5g	10g
Parsnip - 1 cup	100	6g	0.5g	1.5g	24g
Pepper - 1 medium	30	2g	0g	1g	8g
Potato - 1 medium	164	4.5g	0g	4g	37g
Pumpkin - 1 medium	30g	0.5g	0g	1g	7.5g
Radish - 1 cup	13	1g	0g	1g	4g
Spinach - 1 cup	7	1g	0g	1g	1g
Squash - 1 cup	18	1g	0g	1.5g	4g
Sweet Potato - 1 med	112	4g	0g	3g	26g
Tomato - 1 medium	22	1.5g	0g	1g	5g
Turnip - 1 medium	34	2g	0g	1g	8g
Watercress - 1 cup	7	0.5g	0g	1g	0g
Zucchini - 1 medium	32	2g	0.5g	2.5g	6.5g

Nutritional Value of Nuts

	Calories	Fiber	Fat	Protein	Carbs
Almonds - 1 cup	823	17.5g	71g	30g	31g
Brazil - 1 cup	920	10g	93g	20g	17g
Cashews - 1 cup	960	4g	76g	28g	44g
Chestnuts - 1 cup	210	2g	2g	4g	44g
Coconut - 1 cup	490	14g	50g	7g	8g
Hazelnuts - 1 cup	720	8g	72g	16g	16g
Macadamia - 1 cup	961	11g	101g	10.5g	18.5g
Peanuts - 1 cup	825	12g	71g	38g	24g
Pecans - 1 cup	760	4g	80g	12g	16g
Pistachios - 1 cup	740	12g	52g	24g	36g
Walnuts - 1 cup	800	8g	80g	20g	16g

Nutritional Value of Seeds

	Calories	Fiber	Fat	Protein	Carbs
Chia - 1 tablespoon	67	5.5g	4.5g	3g	0.5g
Flax - 1 tablespoon	37	2g	2g	1.5g	2g
Hemp - 1 tablespoon	57	0.5g	4.5g	3.5g	0.5g
Linseeds - 1 tablespoon	49	2.5g	4g	1.5g	2.5g
Poppy - 1 tablespoon	47	1g	4g	1.5g	2g
Pumpkin - 1 tablespoon	56	0.5g	5g	3g	1g
Sesame - 1 tablespoon	52	1g	4.5g	1.5g	2g
Sunflower - 1 tablespoon	47	1g	4g	1.5g	2g

Nutritional Value of Pulses

	Calories	Fiber	Fat	Protein	Carbs
Blackeyed peas - 1 cup	200	8g	4g	12g	34g
Black beans - 1 cup	240	12g	1g	14g	46g
Broad beans - 1 cup	160	8g	0.5g	10g	28g
Butter beans - 1 cup	200	10g	0g	10g	38g
Chickpeas - 1 cup	210	7g	3g	11g	34g
Green Peas - 1 cup	117	7.5g	0.5g	8g	21g
Lentils - 1 cup	320	44g	0g	40g	80g
Mung beans - 1 cup	600	33g	1.5g	49g	110g
Pinto beans - 1 cup	670	30g	2.5g	41g	120g
Kidney beans - 1 cup	216	15.5g	0g	14g	43g
Soya beans - 1 cup	290	12g	14.5g	28g	10g
Split Peas - 1 cup	440	48g	0g	40g	112g

Nutritional Value of Misc

	Calories	Fiber	Fat	Protein	Carbs
Almond milk - 1 cup	60	0.5g	2.5g	0.5g	8g
Almond butter - 1 tbsp	102	0.5g	9g	3.5g	3g
Honey - 1 tbsp	70	0.5g	0g	0g	17g
Soya milk - 1 cup	132	1.5g	4.5g	8g	15.5g
Low-fat yoghurt - 1 cup	125	0g	2.5g	7g	19g
Low-fat milk - 1 cup	110	0g	2.5g	9g	13g
Protein powder - 1 tbsp	110	0g	1.5g	23g	1g
Peanut butter - 1 tbsp	94	1g	8g	4g	3g
Cinnamon - 1 teaspoon	6	1g	0g	0g	4g
Turmeric - 1 tbsp	24	1.5g	0.5g	1g	120g
Oats - 1 cup	166	4g	3.5g	6g	28g
Cod liver oil - 1 tbsp	135	0g	15g	0g	0g
Olive oil - 1 tbsp	120	0g	14g	0g	0g

Conversion Charts

Converting Liquid

US Cups	Metric	Imperial
1 cup	250 ml	8 fl oz
3/4 cup	180 ml	6 fl oz
2/3 cup	150 ml	5 fl oz
1/2 cup	120 ml	4 fl oz
1/3 cup	75 ml	2 1/2 fl oz
1/4 cup	60 ml	2 fl oz
1/8 cup	30 ml	1 fl oz
1 tablespoon	15 ml	1/2 fl oz
1 teaspoon	5 ml	1/6 fl oz

Converting Weight

US Cups	Metric	Imperial
1 cup	150 g	5 oz
3/4 cup	110 g	3 2/3 oz
2/3 cup	100 g	3 1/2 oz
1/2 cup	75 g	2 1/2 oz
1/3 cup	50 g	1 3/4 oz
1/4 cup	40 g	1 1/2 oz
1/8 cup	20 g	3/4 oz
1 tablespoon	10 g	1/3 oz
1 teaspoon	3 g	1/10 oz

Index

135

E

Egg 12, 19, 23, 24, 47, 61, 64, 72, 81
  Noodles 93
  Scrambled 16

F

Falafel 84
Fennel 63, 74, 93
Fish
  Fillets 74
  Sauce 80
  Stock cube 74
Fish cakes 78
Flour 66
  Almond 23, 123
  Plain 95
Frittata 64
Fromage frais 106

G

Garam masala 38, 59
Garlic 12, 19, 21, 31, 42, 57, 59, 60, 65, 66, 68, 69, 77, 82, 89, 107
Gelatin 108
Gelatin water 126
Ginger 28, 33, 59, 65, 66, 78, 88, 97, 98
Granola 22, 108
Green beans 58, 61
Green peas 33

H

Haddock 17
Ham 16, 18
Hazelnuts 111
Honey 14, 22, 25, 114, 119, 123, 125
Hotpot 60

Greek 59

www.ingramcontent.com/pod-product-compliance
Lightning Source LLC
Chambersburg PA
CBHW050134280326
41933CB00010B/1367